The Truth Behind COVID-19 Preview

By: Mack "Cordell" Moore

While every precaution has been taken in the preparation of this book, the publisher assumes no responsibility for errors or omissions, or for damages resulting from the use of the information contained herein.

Plandemic: The Truth Behind Covid-19 Preview

First edition. February 4, 2021.

ISBN: 978-1-716-16987-8

Written by Mack "Cordell" Moore.

Table of Contents

Introduction

I assume most of you are at least aware of the Illuminati or what I prefer to call it, the Antichrist Movement which has been going on for many centuries at least. In case you are not, then I will explain. The Illuminati are a small group of powerful people who control the world. When I mean control, I mean governments, world leaders, religious leaders, organized religion, police and military, banking, wall street, Hollywood, entertainment industry, sports, organized crime, street gangs, drug cartels, porn, sex trafficking, medical industry, corporations, Boule, Knights Templar, Freemasonry, eastern stars, fraternities, sororities, all hate groups, like the KKK, all so-called black groups, etc.

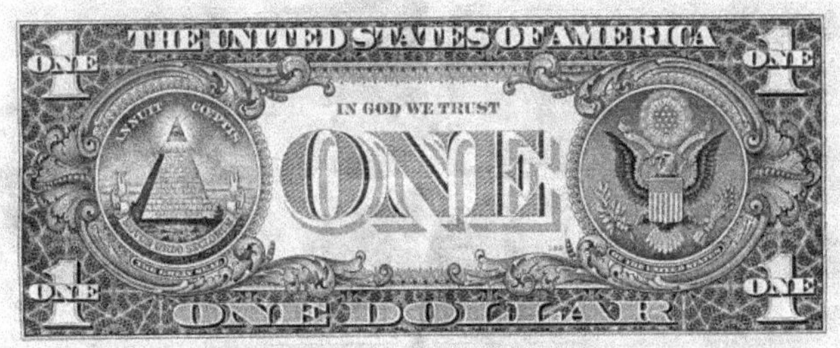

(Image by Hana Chramostova)

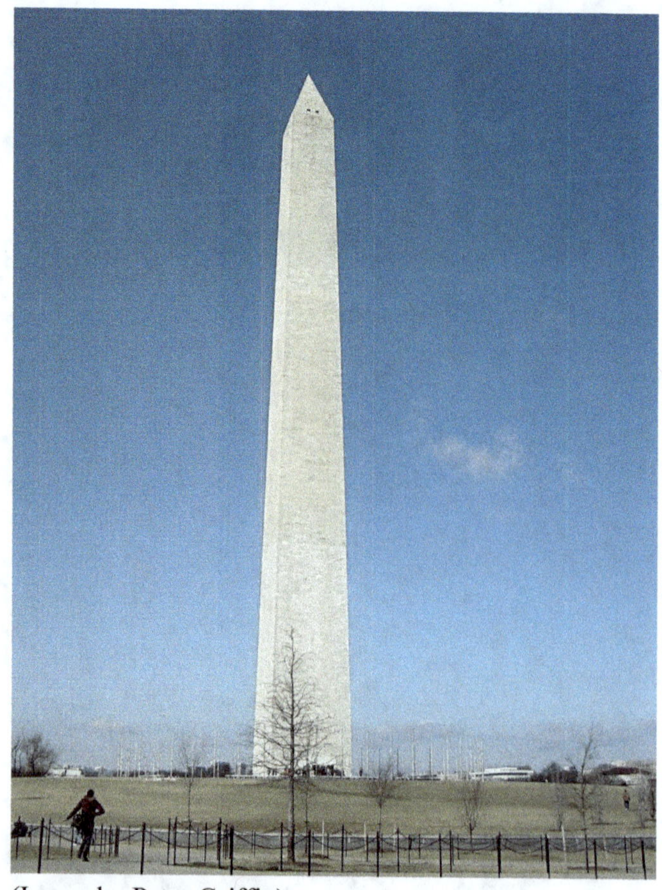

(Image by Peter Griffin)

If we live in America, then why are we
paying homage to the idol gods (demons) of
Ancient Egypt? They designed the
Washington monument after an obelisk and

there is a pyramid on the back of the $1 bill. Ephesians 6:12: "For we wrestle not against flesh and blood, but against principalities, against powers, against the rulers of the darkness of this world, against spiritual wickedness in high places." The real enemies are fallen angels (demons) led by Satan (Lucifer). He gives the Illuminati its power. So truthers can say families like the Rothschilds, or Rockefeller's, or George Soros, but, the devil and his demons, the genuine power behind it all.

People, Christ, will end Satan in due time. Revelation 20:10: "And the devil that deceived them was cast into the lake of fire and brimstone, where the beast and the false prophet are, and shall be tormented day and night for ever and ever." I will go more in depth in the next book.

Vaccine Law & Edom

Coming in 2021 will be a book that exposes the COVID-19 pandemic. What if I told you they planned the Coronavirus pandemic? Would you believe me? Would you just simply dismiss it as the rantings of a crazy conspiracy theorist? What if I could provide proof? Would you be open to hearing me out? Check this out!

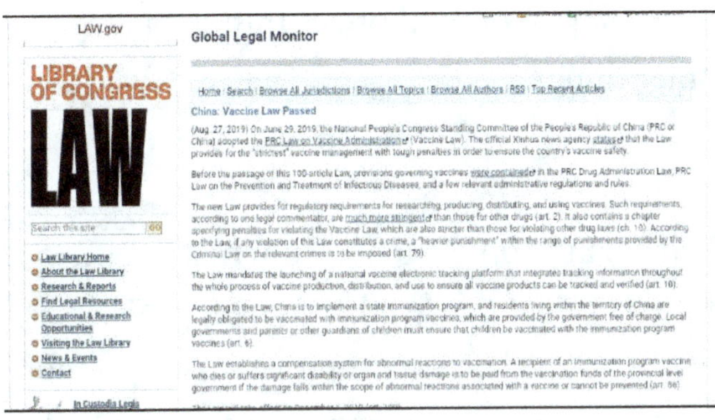

LAW.gov

Global Legal Monitor

Home | Search | Browse All Jurisdictions | Browse All Topics | Browse All Authors | RSS | Top Recent Articles

China: Vaccine Law Passed

(Aug. 27, 2019) On June 29, 2019, the National People's Congress Standing Committee of the People's Republic of China (PRC or China) adopted the PRC Law on Vaccine Administration (Vaccine Law). The official Xinhua news agency states that the Law provides for the "strictest" vaccine management with tough penalties in order to ensure the country's vaccine safety.

Before the passage of this 100-article Law, provisions governing vaccines were contained in the PRC Drug Administration Law, PRC Law on the Prevention and Treatment of Infectious Diseases, and a few relevant administrative regulations and rules.

The new Law provides for regulatory requirements for researching, producing, distributing, and using vaccines. Such requirements, according to one legal commentator, are much more stringent than those for other drugs (art. 2). It also contains a chapter specifying penalties for violating the Vaccine Law, which are also stricter than those for violating other drug laws (ch. 10). According to the Law, if any violation of this Law constitutes a crime, a "heavier punishment" within the range of punishments provided by the Criminal Law on the relevant crimes is to be imposed (art. 79).

The Law mandates the launching of a national vaccine electronic tracking platform that integrates tracking information throughout the whole process of vaccine production, distribution, and use to ensure all vaccine products can be tracked and verified (art. 10).

According to the Law, China is to implement a state immunization program, and residents living within the territory of China are legally obligated to be vaccinated with immunization program vaccines, which are provided by the government free of charge. Local governments and parents or other guardians of children must ensure that children be vaccinated with the immunization program vaccines (art. 6).

The Law establishes a compensation system for abnormal reactions to vaccination. A recipient of an immunization program vaccine who dies or suffers significant disability or organ and tissue damage is to be paid from the vaccination funds of the provincial level government if the damage falls within the scope of abnormal reactions associated with a vaccine or cannot be prevented (art. 56)

LIBRARY OF CONGRESS

LAW

Search this site [GO]

- Law Library Home
- About the Law Library
- Research & Reports
- Find Legal Resources
- Educational & Research Opportunities
- Visiting the Law Library
- News & Events
- Contact

In Custodia Legis

(Source: Library of Congress)

Did you see that? It is a headline from a legit news article about China passing a mandatory vaccine law months before the Coronavirus outbreak. They date the article Aug. 27, 2019, and it is from the Library of Congress. So, it is not from a "conspiracy" source, but a so-called mainstream media source. Why would China pass a vaccine law if there is no outbreak? See, this was a planned epidemic, hence why we in conspiracy circles call it a plandemic. However, some foolishly believe this is a China virus. No, it is not, and hopefully, my upcoming book will prove this and many other things.

What can people expect from this book? Expect to see things like Q-anon get exposed for the psych-op that it is. Look for Donald Trump being exposed for the devil worshipper that he is. Expect to see the Black Lives Matter movement exposed and connected to COVID-19 in ways many of you do not even realize.

For starters, there is no such thing as race. Yes, this is true. The concept of race is used to keep certain people from learning the truth. People are misidentified with race. According to the Word of God, we all have original names and groupings that the devil and his Illuminati does not want us to know. Why? Because then people will learn hidden truths such as the Nation of Edom. Edom exists, but it goes by unique races today. Why is this important? If people knew who the nation of Edom was, then they would know who the real Israelites are.

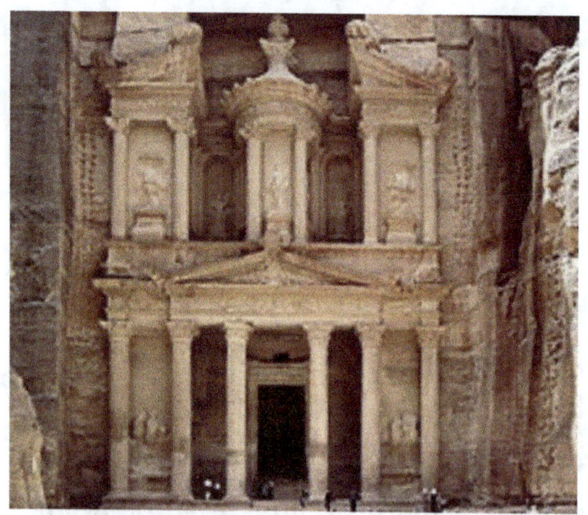

(Source: Wikipedia)

Petra on Mt. Seir is an actual place with what used to be the home of the nation of Edom. The Most High punished them. While some of you reading this may not believe in the bible, Petra is an actual place and featured in certain films. My book will explain who the people of Edom are today and why it's important for all people to know this.

Yes, the people calling themselves Jews are not the real Israelites. Expect some of them, with others, funded and even started the BLM movement. It is for a specific purpose and explained in the upcoming book. What people should pay attention to is not the Anthem protests, but a specific tweet NFL WR DeSean Jackson made which had these fake Jews in an uproar. I will explain it in my book, but in the meantime, you can Google it.

Cell Towers Emit Radiation

This plandemic was ushered in for three major reasons: (1) to ban Christians from gathering to worship, (2) to clear the streets to finish setting up the 5G network, and (3) to force vaccinations on the world's population. Don't believe 5G is a problem? Check this out:

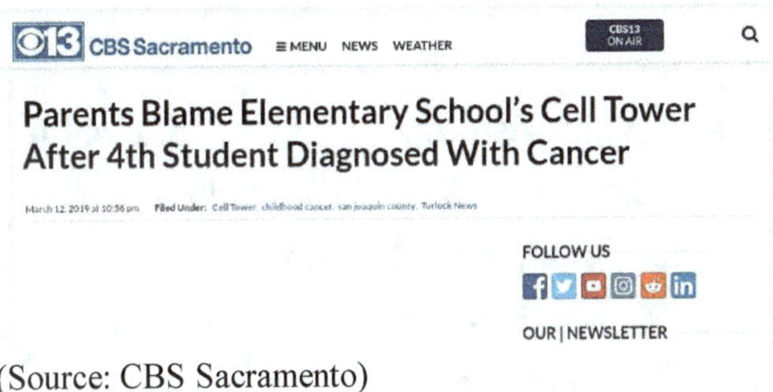

(Source: CBS Sacramento)

The headline is from an article, dated Mar. 2, 2019, in which four schoolchildren got cancer from the radiation emanating from cell towers near Weston Elementary School in Ripon, CA. Yes, all the G's from 1-5G emit harmful radiation which affects us health wise. 5G is the worst of them all. Yes, I will bring it up in more detail in my book so people can know the truth which the Illuminati wants to hide from the public. They even covered this story in Newsweek. There are perhaps more even children diagnosed with cancer from this cell tower. The cell tower is from Sprint and since moved to another spot.

What the masses do not realize is the whole "COVID-19 Pandemic," is mostly a fear tactic to convince people to take the vaccines, which is part of the actual threat. The 5G towers and the vaccines are the genuine threats in all of this. Psalm 91:3: "Surely he shall deliver thee from the snare of the fowler, and from the noisome pestilence (plague/disease)." Matthew 10:28: "And fear not them which kill the body, but are not able to kill the soul: but rather fear him which is able to destroy both soul and body in hell."

What is sad is most of us Christians are being fearful, worrying, and in a panic. We know Christ, who has power over life and death. We shouldn't be fearful or worrying about anything. Philippians 4:6-7: "(6) Be careful for nothing; but in every thing by prayer and supplication with thanksgiving let your requests be made known unto God. (7) And the peace of God, which passeth all understanding, shall keep your hearts and minds through Christ Jesus." 1 Timothy 1:7: "For God hath not given us the spirit of fear; but of power, and of love, and of a sound mind."

We Christians should only fear the Almighty God. If we genuinely believe in Christ, then we shouldn't fear death since we have eternal life through faith in the Savior. We should be willing to die for Jesus because He died for us. My point: we should risk our lives to encourage others, witness to the unsaved, and other things to serve Jesus. Yet we are acting like the world and are in a panic over a disease that's less harmful than Satan's media is portraying.

Note: they derive media from the term Medea. Medea is the goddess (demon) of illusion. The media are under the influence of the fallen angel Lucifer (Satan). Do we Christians not discern the evil spirits influencing the media when they discuss the Covid pandemic? God did not give us the spirit of fear. However, Satan sends this spirit, and others, like worry, panic, chaos, confusion, anxiety, amongst others, to attack saved and unsaved alike.

Empty Hospitals & Layoffs

I will admit it. I worried and panicked when all this started. However, seeking Christ by prayer, fasting, and reading His Word has eased those concerns. The Holy Spirit has calmed my nerves and He will do the same for you if you ask Him. Did you know in certain places they laid off hospital workers?

Mercy reveals scope of workforce cuts in St. Louis: 204 layoffs, 459 furloughs

In a letter to the state, Mercy said 204 workers would be laid off in St. Louis and another 459 would be furloughed

(Source: ksdk.com)

The headline is from May 26, 2020, discussing how they laid off or furloughed several hundred healthcare workers from Mercy hospital in the St. Louis area. Some were doctors and some were nurses. These types of layoffs have been happening across the United States. If we are in a pandemic, then why are nurses and doctors being laid off? Don't overcrowded hospitals need the staff? This is a lie! Hospitals are less crowded than what the reports say.

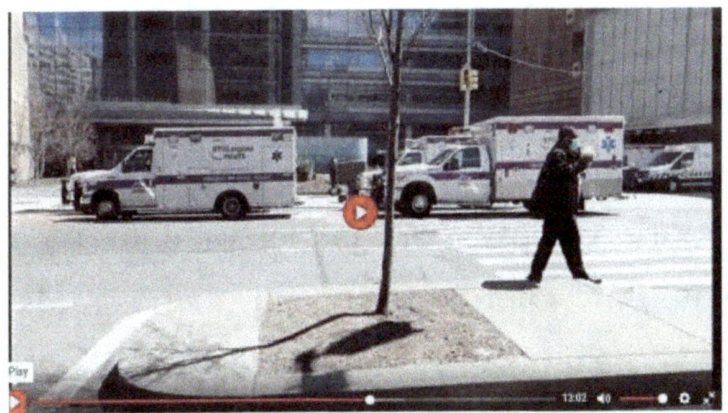

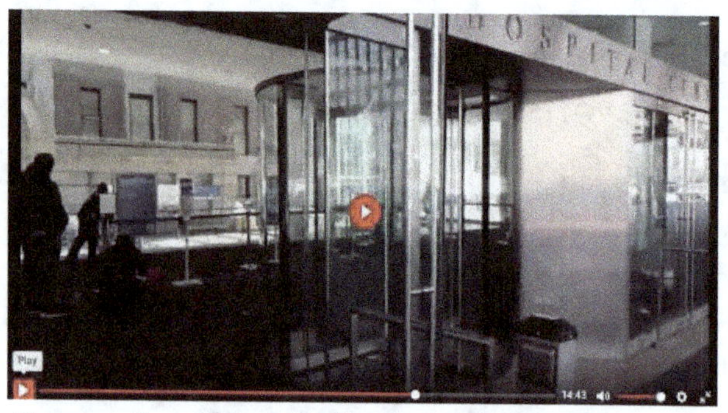

(Source: Sananvapaus Channel on Bitchute)

The 1st image is the outside entrance of Tisch Hospital in New York. The second image is of the lobby of Bellevue Hospital in New York. If New York is the epicenter of the pandemic, then why are 2 of its hospitals appear to be empty? YouTube has removed many vids exposing this. Hospitals aren't just empty in New York, but other states like Colorado and Washington to name a few. You can find this out on the site called Bitchute. I am a YouTuber and have had certain vids removed that expose certain truths, like the Las Vegas Shooting, for example. It was a staged event. No one died, but the media lied about it being an actual shooting.

This is what YouTube does. Try to hinder certain truths from getting out. I could write an entire book about how YouTube and all social media sites are trying to censor the truth from getting out, but I digress. What I will say YouTube is guilty of enabling underground pedo rings on its site. Please research and learn more about it!

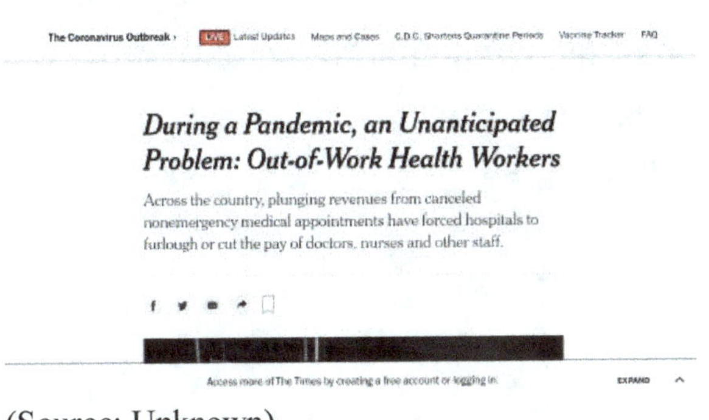

(Source: Unknown)

This is a headline from April 3, 2020. I suggest you all read the article. To sum it up, healthcare workers in New York and other places like Nevada, Washington, D.C., Detroit, and other places got laid off, or furloughed, or reassigned, or took pay cuts. Their reasoning is allegedly these hospitals need staff trained to deal with the pandemic. So, they don't need other specialists. I am not buying it. If you look back at the pics of the empty Hospitals and parked Ambulances, then there is no real outbreak. Note: hospitals are just like any corporation and they all profit from layoffs. Hospitals are using this plandemic to increase profits through layoffs, pay cuts, and furloughs. Think about it, people.

Bill Gates & Vaccines

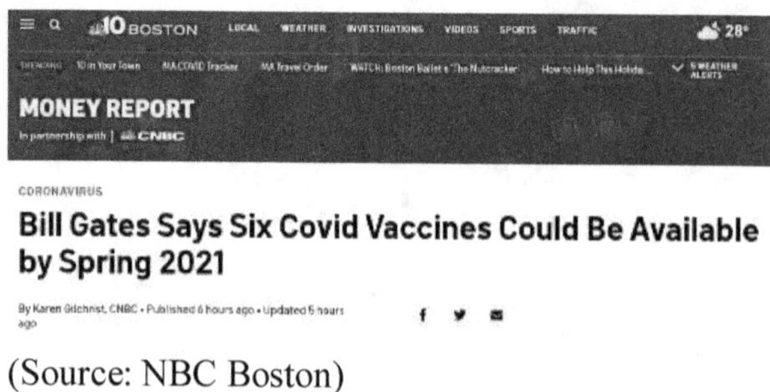

(Source: NBC Boston)

There is no way I was not going to at least mention Bill Gates. The headline is from a recent NBC Boston article in which Mr. Gates is promising six vaccines by spring of 2021. He has companies such as Pfizer and Johnson & Johnson set and ready to go. Bill Gates is funding a vaccine to help people. Does he want to help people? Or does he have ulterior motives? Question: why don't the public have any problem with this? If he can't fix or solve computer viruses, then how is he qualified to handle a biological virus? It is not like he has a medical degree.

Now I know detractors will say he isn't the one making the vaccine but funding the project. On that you are correct. Question: has he publicly said he would take the vaccine? I don't believe he would. My point: challenge him to put his money where his mouth is. If he is so sure vaccines are safe, then he should be the first in line to take them. He should vaccinate his children. If not, then this would be a pause for concern.

He sure seems in a big hurry to roll out these vaccines. Have they tested them? Have the FDA carefully approved the vaccines? Then again, the FDA will rush to approve anything. Just examine Lucky Charms, for example. Tri sodium phosphate is a chemical believed to be in paint thinner. Some may dispute this, but it is also used as a cleaning agent found in stain removers, soaps, and detergents.

Is it safe for us to consume something used to remove stains? No. I would challenge anyone to look up the products we buy and learn the chemicals they put in them. They are poisoning us. The weed killer Roundup causes cancer, yet the FDA also approved it. How can we be sure these vaccines are safe?

APRIL 23, 2020

The Bill Gates Effect: WHO's DTP Vaccine Killed More Children in Africa Than the Diseases it Targeted

By Robert F. Kennedy, Jr.

(Source: Children's Health Defense)

This article, from Robert Kennedy, Jr. alleges that Bill Gates' DTP vaccine killed thousands of children in Africa. It's an interesting article. Perhaps take it with a grain of salt. I believe there's truth in the article. It claims that girls who took the vaccine died at a rate 10 times higher than unvaccinated children. The vaccine compromised the immune systems of all children who took it.

Do we know what is in vaccines? Allegedly mercury, aluminum, formaldehyde, and other harmful things. The government-owned science community will tell you that formaldehyde is safe. Yeah, right! They use the same formaldehyde in embalming fluid. The same embalming fluid some people foolishly lace with marijuana to get high.

Anti-Vaccine Doctor Dies Mysteriously

(Source: Washington Post)

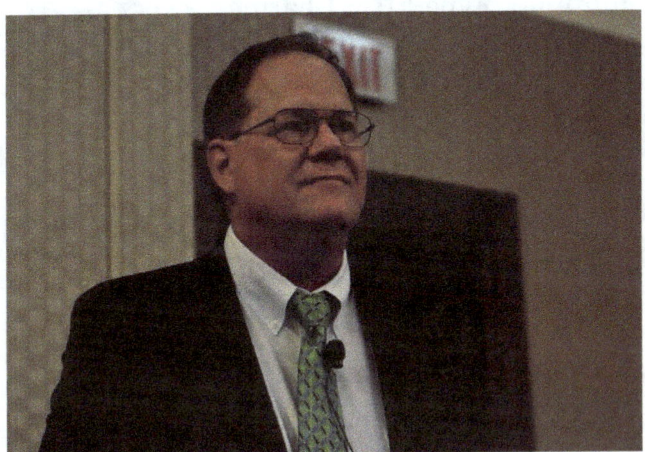

(Image Courtesy of Washington Post)

Dr. James Bradstreet was an actual medical doctor who was against vaccinations. He died mysteriously in 2015. The C.I.A. owned Washington Post did an article mocking Dr. Bradstreet in the headline about an autism "cure" he was peddling. My thoughts: the Washington Post's article on Bradstreet is just a C.I.A. plot to discredit him and his work. His death ruled a suicide, but I believe they murdered him because of a protein (GcMAF) treatment he was providing people which goes against Illuminati owned Big Pharma.

There are dozens of holistic doctors who were treating people with GcMAF, and they all died mysteriously. Their Google, their doctors, their Big Pharma, their media, etc. will tell you how GcMAF protein is harmful and the harmful products they peddle are safe. Keep in mind the FDA still approves of cigarettes known to cause things like lung cancer, emphysema, etc. Cigarettes are just as addictive as any illegal drugs out there, yet those are still legal to buy and use. Note: the government belongs to Satan, who hates humanity, so it does not care about people's health. They care more about making profits.

Bradstreet's death was a gunshot wound to the chest, yet the gun was not on his person, but "nearby" in the water. He didn't kill himself just like Epstein did not kill himself. Bradstreet testified twice before Congress speaking against vaccines and the Illuminati owned Feds raided his offices the day before his "suicide." They did this to discredit him. By the way, GcMAF, not approved by the FDA, yet as I mentioned, they approve dangerous products all the time. So, it is not a safety issue, but a profit issue in part. Big Pharma possibly wanted to protect its profits, so a doctor promoting an autism "cure" had to go. This is my belief. Who makes the vaccines? Big Pharma and if the vaccines are obsolete, then no profits. Think about it!

Don't take the vaccines! It's a trap! I know I won't be. They will find it much easier to kill me than to get me to take their vaccines. For one, it is believed the vaccines have the mark of the beast (666) in them. Revelation 13:16-18: "(16) 16 And he causeth all, both small and great, rich and poor, free and bond, to receive a mark in their right hand, or in their foreheads: (17) And that no man might buy or sell, save he that had the mark, or the name of the beast, or the number of his name. (18) Here is wisdom. Let him that hath understanding count the number of the beast: for it is the number of a man; and his number is Six hundred threescore and six."

I believe this vaccine is a precursor of the mark of the beast, but not the actual mark. I believe the something added to the vaccine will have 666 on it. What is that something? You must read my book to find out. What I will say is this, it is connected to QAnon. As for the mark of the beast, the False Prophet (second beast) will be the one as mentioned in Rev. 13:16 who causes unbelievers from all walks of life (rich and poor) to wear the mark which will be in their right hand or foreheads. This mark will be 666 or the name of the Antichrist. The last time I checked, they will inject the vaccines inside a person's arm.

Conclusion

Well, this is where I am about to cut it short. I hope I have you salivating for the actual book. Matthew 5:13: "Ye are the salt of the earth: but if the salt have lost his savour, wherewith shall it be salted? it is thenceforth good for nothing, but to be cast out, and to be trodden under foot of men." Christ calls for His true followers to be salts of the earth to draw unbelievers to seek Christ, the only way to heaven. Christ, then gives new believers the Living Water (Holy Spirit) to quench our spiritual thirst.

Think of my upcoming book as a sermon with conspiracies and other facts mixed in. There will be plenty to cover. I will highlight; George Floyd and perhaps Breonna Taylor to explain how those incidents were "staged" or at least raise doubts in the minds of people about the validity of these stories. Make no mistake, profiling and police brutality happens, mainly to my people, but to others as well. However, the actual stories hardly become national stories. I got harassed by police before, but they staged an incident like George Floyd, for example, to increase the tension that is already there. Remember my people are ⅗ of a man according to the Constitution. There is a reasoning for it, and I will explain it in the upcoming book.

(Source: New York Post)

I wanted to share the image of the headline from newyorkpost.com highlighting CBS

News using footage from Italy claiming it is from an NYC hospital. According to Fox News, it was an honest mistake. I revealed to you earlier that NY hospitals were empty. Yes, people can make honest mistakes, but in this case, they did it on purpose to help create mass hysteria and panic. The Illuminati owned media tells a narrative which may not always be truthful. My belief: the media lies often.

I want to encourage all people, especially true Christians throughout the world, reminding them the Messiah (Jesus Christ) is always in control. He has the power to heal all diseases if it is His will. We have eternal life even if He allows us to die. Why are we worried over this? We should show complete faith in Christ that He will help us no matter what.

One last thing: don't take the vaccines under any circumstances! They are trying to scare us into taking them, which should raise eyebrows. The medical industry is under the Illuminati's control. To become doctors, people must disobey the Most High by taking the Hippocratic oath. James 5:12: "But above all things, my brethren, swear not, neither by heaven, neither by the earth, neither by any other oath: but let your yea be yea; and your nay, nay; lest ye fall into condemnation." Just like freemasons, eastern stars, fraternities, and sororities, doctors take oaths that the Word of God forbids.

Even the logo for the American Medical Association is evil, but I will expound on it in the upcoming book. Just like how the word pharmacy got derived from a term that has evil roots behind it. What do I mean? You will find this out and more in 2021.

Thanks for reading and be sure to leave a review to show this author support.

Cordell's Other Books

Be sure to check out my other books!

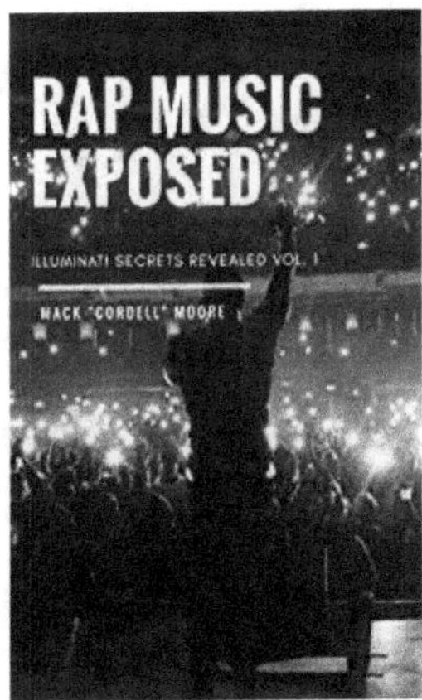

Rap Music Exposed

The 1st book in the Illuminati Secrets Revealed Series which explores the dark side of hip-hop!

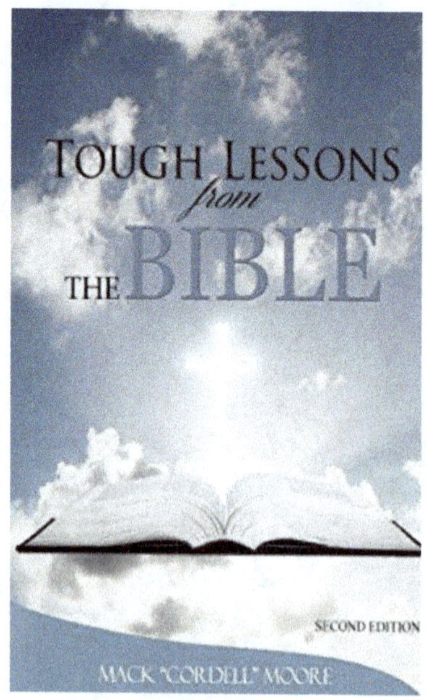

Tough Lessons from the Bible

A book on certain bible study topics such as homosexuality, and the pagan origins of Christmas!

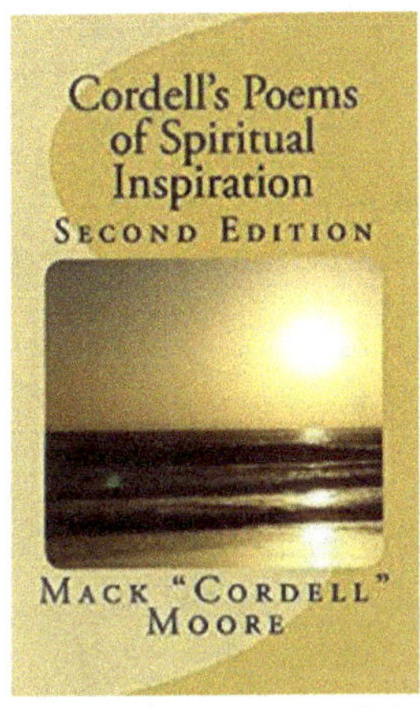

Cordell's Poems of Spiritual Inspiration

This book is a collection of inspirational poems that encourages those who are depressed and feeling suicidal!

Mack's Amazon Author Page:

(www.amazon.com/Mack-Cordell-Moore/e/B00I8ZK6CQ/)

Follow me on Social Media:

Instagram
(https://www.instagram.com/illuminati_secrets_r
evealed)

Facebook
(https://www.facebook.com/Cordell.79)

Twitter
(https://twitter.com/Cordell_79)

YouTube
(https://www.youtube.com/Illuminati_Secrets_Revealed)

Bitchute
(www.bitchute.com/channel/Illuminati_Secrets_revealed
)

I.S.R. Website
(http://www.illuminatisecretsrevealed.com)

Illuminati Secrets Revealed Store

(https://www.teespring.com/stores/illuminati-secrets-revealed)

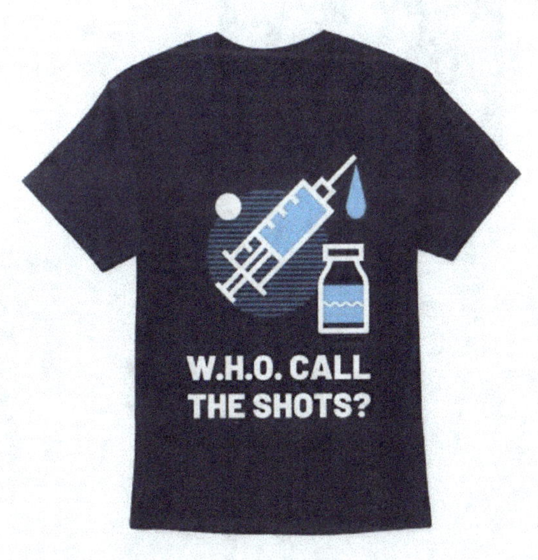

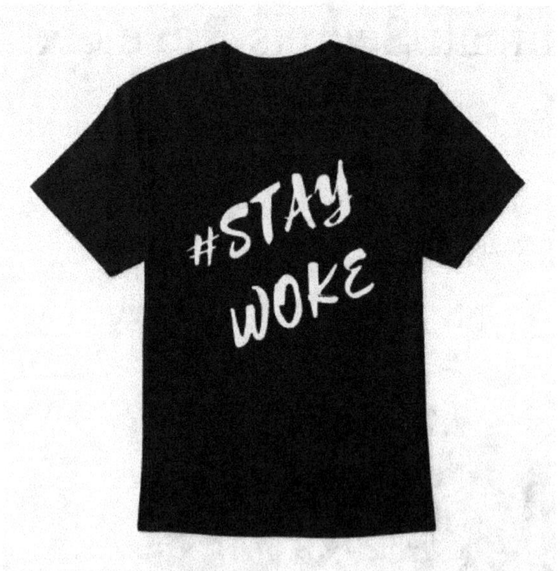
#STAY
WOKE

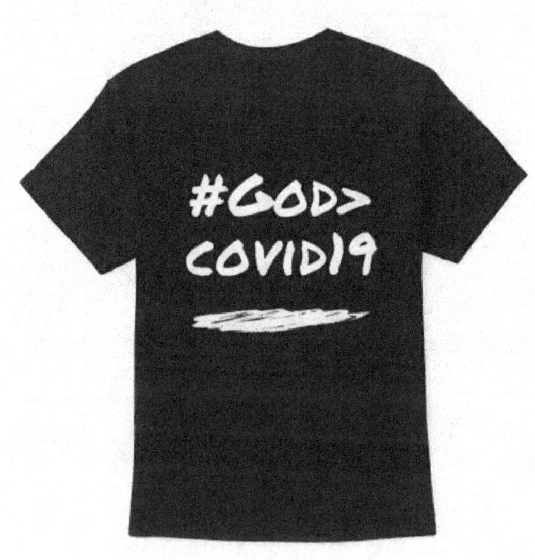

Get 30% off on anything you buy by using this coupon code at checkout: WOKE